The Easy PCOS Diet Cookbook

Hormone Balancing Insulin Resistance Recipes Meal Plan and Fertility Nutrition for Busy Individuals

Dr. Olivia Tastewell

TABLE OF CONTENTS

INTRODUCTION

AGNES HAD POLYCYSTIC OVARY syndrome (PCOS), a hormonal disorder that affects millions of women worldwide. She had been struggling with it for years, ever since she was diagnosed at the age of 18. She had tried everything to manage her symptoms, from birth control pills to metformin to supplements. But nothing seemed to work. She felt like she was fighting a losing battle. She knew that diet and lifestyle changes were important for PCOS, but she didn't know where to start. She was overwhelmed by the conflicting information on the internet, the fad diets, and the expensive products.

She didn't have the time or the energy to cook complicated meals or count calories or carbs. She needed something simple, easy, and effective. One day, she was having lunch with her coworker, who also had PCOS. Her coworker looked radiant, happy, and confident. She had lost weight, cleared her skin, and improved her mood. She had also gotten pregnant after years of trying. Agnes was curious and asked her what her secret was.

Her coworker smiled and handed her a copy of this book. She said that it was the best thing that ever happened to her. She said that it changed her life. This book is not just a cookbook. It is a guide to hormone balancing, insulin resistance, and fertility nutrition for busy individuals with PCOS. It is based on the latest scientific research and the experience of thousands of women who have successfully reversed their PCOS symptoms naturally.

This book will show you how to balance your hormones, lower your insulin levels, and boost your fertility with delicious and nutritious recipes. You will learn how to choose the best foods for PCOS and avoid the worst ones.

You will discover how to make easy, quick, and satisfying meals for every occasion, from breakfast to dinner, from dessert to snack, from smoothie to side dish. You will also find out how to customize your diet according to your preferences, goals, and needs. This book is for you if you want to take control of your PCOS and your health. You want to eat well without spending hours in the kitchen or breaking the bank. You want to feel good in your body and your mind. You want to get pregnant or improve your chances of conceiving. You want to join a community of supportive and inspiring women who are on the same journey as you.

This book is not for you if you are looking for a magic pill or a quick fix. You are not willing to make any changes to your diet or lifestyle. You are not interested in learning about the science behind PCOS and nutrition. You are not ready to embrace your power and your potential.

If you are ready to transform your PCOS and your life, then this book is for you. It is time to stop suffering and start living. It is time to reclaim your health and your happiness. It is time to discover the easy PCOS diet cookbook.

Protein Waffles

Protein waffles provide a balanced breakfast with a good mix of protein, healthy fats from peanut butter, and natural sugars from bananas. This can help regulate blood sugar levels and support hormone balance.

Ingredients:
- Frozen protein waffles (2 waffles)
- Peanut butter (to taste)
- Banana (1, sliced)

Serving Size:
2 waffles
Cooking Time:
5 minutes
Instructions:
1. Toast the frozen protein waffles according to package instructions.
2. Spread a layer of peanut butter on each waffle.
3. Top with sliced bananas.
4. Enjoy your protein-packed and PCOS-friendly breakfast!

Yogurt Bowl

Greek yogurt provides a good source of protein, and the combination of nut butter, granola, and berries adds a variety of nutrients. This can help manage weight and support overall health in PCOS patients.

Ingredients:
- Greek yogurt (1 cup)
- Nut butter (1 tablespoon)
- Granola (1/4 cup)
- Berries (1/2 cup)

Serving Size:
1 bowl
Cooking Time:
5 minutes

Instructions:
1. Take a bowl and put some Greek yogurt in it.
2. Drizzle with your favorite nut butter.
3. Sprinkle granola on top.
4. Add a handful of fresh berries.
5. Mix it all for a delicious yogurt bowl.

Protein Oats

Oatmeal is a complex carbohydrate, and when combined with protein powder, nuts, and fruit, it provides sustained energy and supports blood sugar control.

Ingredients:
- Oatmeal (1/2 cup)
- Whole milk (1 cup)
- Protein powder (1 scoop)
- Chopped nuts (2 tablespoons)
- Fruit of your choice (1/2 cup, chopped)

Serving Size:
1 bowl
Cooking Time:
10 minutes

Instructions:
1. Cook oatmeal with whole milk according to package instructions.
2. Stir in your preferred protein powder.
3. Top with chopped nuts and fresh fruit.
4. Mix well and enjoy a hearty and PCOS-friendly bowl of protein oats.

Cereal Bowl

This cereal bowl provides a balance of protein, fiber, and healthy fats, promoting satiety and helping manage blood sugar levels in PCOS patients.

Ingredients:
- Protein/fiber cereal (1 cup)
- Whole milk or alternative (1 cup)
- Turkey bacon (2 slices, cooked and crumbled)
- Nuts (2 tablespoons)
- Fruit (1/2 cup)

Serving Size:
1 bowl
Cooking Time:
5 minutes

Instructions:
1. Pour the protein/fiber cereal into a bowl.
2. Add whole milk or your preferred alternative.
3. Top with crumbled turkey bacon, nuts, and fresh fruit.
4. Mix well and enjoy a nutritious cereal bowl.

Green Smoothie

The green smoothie offers a nutrient-dense option with Greek yogurt, spinach, and flaxseed, providing essential vitamins and minerals for PCOS patients.

Ingredients:
- Greek yogurt or kefir (1 cup)
- Frozen fruit (1 cup)
- Spinach (1 cup)
- Flaxseed (1 tablespoon)
- Avocado (1/2)

Serving Size:
1 smoothie
Cooking Time:
5 minutes

Instructions:
1. In a blender, combine Greek yogurt or kefir, frozen fruit, spinach, flaxseed, and avocado.
2. Blend until smooth.
3. Pour into a glass and enjoy a nourishing and PCOS-friendly green smoothie.

Bento Box

The bento box offers a variety of nutrients from boiled eggs, yogurt, nuts, and fruits, providing a balanced and satisfying breakfast.

Ingredients:
- Boiled eggs (2)
- Yogurt (1/2 cup)
- Nuts (2 tablespoons)
- Fruit (1/2 cup)
- Cucumber (sliced)
- Muffin (1, optional)

Serving Size:
1 bento box
Cooking Time:
10 minutes

Instructions:
1. Place boiled eggs, yogurt, nuts, fruit, cucumber slices, and a muffin (if desired) in a bento box.
2. Enjoy this diverse and PCOS-friendly breakfast with a bit of everything!

Quick Breakfast Cup

This quick breakfast cup provides a convenient and balanced option with Greek yogurt, nut/granola bar, and banana, offering a mix of protein, fiber, and natural sugars for sustained energy and blood sugar control.

Ingredients:
- Greek yogurt cup (1)
- Nut/granola bar (1)
- Banana (1, sliced)

Serving Size:
1 serving
Cooking Time:
No cooking required

Instructions:
1. Simply open the Greek yogurt cup.
2. Pair it with a nut or granola bar.
3. Add sliced banana on top.
4. Mix if desired and enjoy.

Homemade Muffin Combo

This homemade muffin combo with boiled eggs and trail mix offers a blend of protein, healthy fats, and complex carbs, providing a satisfying and balanced breakfast for PCOS patients.

Ingredients:
- Homemade muffin (1)
- Boiled eggs (2)
- Trail mix (1/4 cup)

Serving Size:
1 serving
Cooking Time:
30 minutes (includes muffin preparation)

Instructions:
1. Prepare homemade muffins in advance.
2. Serve with boiled eggs and a portion of trail mix.
3. Enjoy a wholesome and PCOS-friendly muffin combo for breakfast.

Baked Egg Cups

Baked egg muffin cups with apple and peanut butter offer a balanced mix of protein, healthy fats, and fiber, supporting blood sugar management and overall well-being in PCOS patients.

Ingredients:
- Baked egg muffins/cups (2)
- Apple (1, sliced)
- Peanut butter (2 tablespoons)

Serving Size:
1 serving
Cooking Time:
20 minutes (includes baking time)

Instructions:
1. Bake or prepare the egg muffins/cups in advance.
2. Serve with sliced apple and a side of peanut butter.
3. Enjoy a tasty and PCOS-friendly breakfast with baked egg cups.

Avocado Toast with Egg

Avocado toast with egg on whole grain bread provides a combination of healthy fats, protein, and complex carbs, offering a satisfying and nutrient-rich breakfast for PCOS patients.

Ingredients:
- Whole grain toast (2 slices)
- Avocado (1/2)
- Egg (1)

Serving Size:
1 serving
Cooking Time:
10 minutes

Instructions:
1. Toast whole grain bread slices.
2. Spread mashed avocado on each slice.
3. Cook an egg as desired (poached, fried, or boiled).
4. Place the egg on top of the avocado toast.
5. Enjoy a delicious and PCOS-friendly avocado toast with egg.

Lunch Recipes

Salmon over Baby Spinach

This recipe provides a nutrient-rich lunch with omega-3 fatty acids from salmon and iron-rich baby spinach, supporting hormonal balance and overall well-being in PCOS patients.

Ingredients:
- Salmon fillet (6 oz)
- Baby spinach (2 cups, fresh)
- Olive oil (1 tablespoon)
- Lemon juice (1 tablespoon)
- Salt and pepper to taste

Serving Size:
1 serving
Cooking Time:
15 minutes

1. Sprinkle a little bit of salt and pepper on the salmon to give it flavor.
2. In a pan, heat olive oil over medium heat.
3. Cook salmon for about 3-4 minutes per side or until fully cooked.
4. Place salmon over a bed of fresh baby spinach.
5. Drizzle with lemon juice.
6. Enjoy a PCOS-friendly lunch with salmon over baby spinach.

Turkey Wrap with Apple

This turkey wraps with an apple provides a balanced meal with lean protein from turkey and fiber from the apple, promoting satiety and aiding blood sugar control in PCOS patients.

Ingredients:
- Turkey slices (4 oz)
- Whole wheat or spinach wrap (1)
- Apple (1, thinly sliced)
- Mustard or Greek yogurt dressing (to taste)

Serving Size:
1 wrap

Cooking Time:
10 minutes

1. Lay the turkey slices on the wrap.
2. Add a thinly sliced apple.
3. Drizzle with mustard or Greek yogurt dressing.
4. Wrap it up and enjoy a PCOS-friendly turkey wrap with apple.

Beet, Goat Cheese, Broccoli Salad

This vibrant salad offers a mix of nutrients from beets, broccoli, and goat cheese, providing fiber and antioxidants that support hormonal balance and overall health in PCOS patients.

Ingredients:
- Cooked beets (1 cup, diced)
- Goat cheese (2 oz, crumbled)
- Broccoli florets (1 cup)
- Mixed greens (2 cups)
- Olive oil (1 tablespoon)
- Balsamic vinegar (1 tablespoon)
- Salt and pepper to taste

Serving Size:
1 serving
Cooking Time:
15 minutes

Instructions:

1. Steam or blanch broccoli florets.
2. In a bowl, combine beets, goat cheese, broccoli, and mixed greens.
3. Drizzle with olive oil and balsamic vinegar.
4. Season with salt and pepper.
5. Toss gently and enjoy a delicious and PCOS-friendly beet, goat cheese, and broccoli salad.

Grab 'n' Go Egg Muffins

These egg muffins are a great source of protein and healthy fats, supporting satiety and blood sugar control in PCOS patients.

Ingredients:

- Eggs (4)

- Spinach (1 cup, chopped)

- Cherry tomatoes (1/2 cup, diced)

- Feta cheese (1/4 cup, crumbled)

- Salt and pepper to taste

Serving Size:

1 serving (2-3 muffins)

Cooking Time:

25 minutes

Instructions:

1. Before you start cooking, warm up the oven to 350°F (175°C).

2. In a bowl, whisk eggs and season with salt and pepper.

3. Add chopped spinach, diced cherry tomatoes, and crumbled feta cheese. Mix well.

4. Pour the mixture into muffin cups.

5. Bake for 20-25 minutes or until eggs are set.

6. Allow to cool and enjoy these PCOS-friendly Grab 'n' Go Egg Muffins.

Swiss Chard Quiche

This Swiss chard quiche provides a combination of protein, vitamins, and minerals, contributing to overall well-being and hormonal balance in PCOS patients.

Ingredients:

- Swiss chard (2 cups, chopped)

- Eggs (4)

- Milk or dairy-free alternative (1 cup)

- Feta cheese (1/2 cup, crumbled)

- Whole wheat pie crust (1, pre-made or homemade)

- Salt and pepper to taste

Serving Size:

1 slice (1/8th of the quiche)

Cooking Time:

45 minutes

1. Before you start cooking, warm up the oven to 375°F (190°C).

2. In a pan, sauté chopped Swiss chard until wilted.

3. In a bowl, whisk eggs and mix with milk, feta cheese, salt, and pepper.

4. Place the pie crust in a quiche pan and add the sautéed Swiss chard.

5. Pour the egg mixture over the chard.

6. Bake for 35-40 minutes or until the center is set.

7. Allow to cool before slicing and enjoy a PCOS-friendly Swiss Chard Quiche.

Asian Chicken Slaw

This Asian chicken slaw offers a protein-rich and low-carb option with fresh vegetables, supporting a balanced diet for PCOS patients.

Ingredients:

- Chicken breast (8 oz, cooked and shredded)

- Napa cabbage (2 cups, shredded)

- Carrots (1 cup, julienned)

- Red bell pepper (1, thinly sliced)

- Snow peas (1/2 cup, sliced)

- Sesame oil (1 tablespoon)

- Soy sauce (2 tablespoons)

- Rice vinegar (1 tablespoon)

- Sesame seeds (1 tablespoon)

Serving Size:

1 serving

Cooking Time:

20 minutes

Instructions:

1. In a bowl, combine shredded chicken, Napa cabbage, julienned carrots, sliced red bell pepper, and sliced snow peas.

2. In a separate bowl, whisk together sesame oil, soy sauce, and rice vinegar.

3. Drizzle the dressing all over the salad and mix it well so that everything gets coated.

4. Sprinkle sesame seeds on top.

5. Enjoy a refreshing and PCOS-friendly Asian Chicken Slaw.

Spinach Chicken Poppers

Spinach chicken poppers provide a lean source of protein from chicken and nutrient-rich spinach, supporting muscle health and overall well-being.

Ingredients:
- Ground chicken (1 lb)
- Spinach (1 cup, chopped)
- Garlic powder (1 teaspoon)
- Onion powder (1 teaspoon)
- Paprika (1/2 teaspoon)
- Salt and pepper to taste

Serving Size:
4 servings
Cooking Time:
20 minutes

Instructions:

1. start heating your oven to 400°F (200°C) before cooking.

2. In a bowl, mix ground chicken, chopped spinach, garlic powder, onion powder, paprika, salt, and pepper.

3. Form the mixture into small poppers and place them on a baking sheet.

4. Put it in the oven and let it cook for 15-20 minutes or until it's completely done.

5. Serve and enjoy these PCOS-friendly Spinach Chicken Poppers.

Chicken Collard Wraps

Chicken collard wraps offer a low-carb alternative to traditional wraps, providing protein from chicken and a variety of nutrients from collard greens.

Ingredients:

- Cooked chicken breast (8 oz, shredded)

- Collard green leaves (4 large)

- Hummus (1/2 cup)

- Cherry tomatoes (1/2 cup, sliced)

- Cucumber (1, julienned)

- Avocado (1, sliced)

Serving Size:

2 wraps

Cooking Time:

15 minutes

Instructions:

1. Lay collard green leaves flat.

2. Spread hummus on each leaf.

3. Add shredded chicken, sliced cherry tomatoes, julienned cucumber, and avocado.

4. Roll up the collard leaves to form wraps.

5. Slice in half and enjoy your Chicken Collard Wraps.

Guacamole Chicken Salad

Guacamole chicken salad provides a good source of healthy fats from avocados, along with lean protein from chicken, supporting hormonal balance and satiety in PCOS patients.

Ingredients:

- Cooked chicken breast (8 oz, diced)

- Avocado (2, mashed)

- Cherry tomatoes (1 cup, halved)

- Red onion (1/4 cup, finely chopped)

- Cilantro (2 tablespoons, chopped)

- Lime juice (2 tablespoons)

- Salt and pepper to taste

Serving Size:
4 servings
Cooking Time:
15 minutes

Instructions:

1. In a bowl, combine diced chicken, mashed avocado, halved cherry tomatoes, chopped red onion, cilantro, lime juice, salt, and pepper.

2. Mix well until ingredients are evenly coated.

3. Serve and enjoy this flavorful and PCOS-friendly Guacamole Chicken Salad.

Sweet Potato Noodle Salad

Sweet potato noodle salad provides complex carbohydrates from sweet potatoes, along with a variety of nutrients, supporting sustained energy and overall health.

Ingredients:

- Sweet potato noodles (2 cups, spiralized)

- Mixed greens (2 cups)

- Cherry tomatoes (1 cup, halved)

- Feta cheese (1/2 cup, crumbled)

- Pecans (1/4 cup, chopped)

- Balsamic vinaigrette dressing (2 tablespoons)

Serving Size:
2 servings
Cooking Time:
15 minutes

Instructions:

1. Cook sweet potato noodles according to package instructions.

2. In a bowl, combine sweet potato noodles, mixed greens, cherry tomatoes, crumbled feta cheese, and chopped pecans.

3. Drizzle with balsamic vinaigrette dressing and toss to combine.

4. Serve and enjoy this delicious Sweet Potato Noodle Salad.

Dinner Recipes

Pulled Pork

Pulled pork is a good source of lean protein, providing essential amino acids for muscle health and aiding in blood sugar control.

Ingredients:
- Pork shoulder or butt (3 lbs)
- BBQ sauce (1 cup)
- Onion (1, sliced)
- Garlic cloves (3, minced)
- Salt and pepper to taste

Serving Size:
6 servings
Cooking Time:
6-8 hours (slow cooker) or 3-4 hours (oven)

Instructions:

1. Use your hands to spread some salt and pepper all over the pork.

2. Place pork in a slow cooker or oven-safe dish.

3. Add sliced onion, minced garlic, and BBQ sauce.

4. Cook on low heat (slow cooker) or 300°F (oven) until the pork is tender and easily shredded.

5. Shred the pork and mix with the sauce.

6. Serve and enjoy this PCOS-friendly Pulled Pork.

Creamy Tomato Baked Fish

Creamy tomato baked fish provides a lean protein source with omega-3 fatty acids, supporting cardiovascular health and hormonal balance in PCOS patients.

Ingredients:
- White fish fillets (4, 6 oz each)
- Tomato sauce (1 cup)
- Greek yogurt or sour cream (1/2 cup)
- Garlic powder (1 teaspoon)
- Dried oregano (1 teaspoon)
- Salt and pepper to taste

Serving Size:
4 servings
Cooking Time:
25 minutes

Instructions:

1. Before you start cooking, warm up the oven to 375°F (190°C).
2. Place fish fillets in a baking dish.
3. In a bowl, mix tomato sauce, Greek yogurt or sour cream, garlic powder, dried oregano, salt, and pepper.
4. Pour the sauce over the fish.
5. Bake for 20-25 minutes or until the fish is cooked through.
6. Serve and enjoy this creamy tomato-baked fish.

Zambrero's Burrito Bowl

Zambrero's burrito bowl provides a customizable option with a balance of protein, healthy fats, and fiber, offering a satisfying and nutritious meal for PCOS patients.

Ingredients:
- Cooked brown rice (2 cups)
- Black beans (1 cup, cooked)
- Grilled chicken or your protein of choice (6 oz)
- Lettuce (1 cup, shredded)
- Tomato salsa (1/2 cup)
- Guacamole (1/4 cup)
- Greek yogurt or sour cream (2 tablespoons)
- Cheese (1/4 cup, shredded)

Serving Size:

1 serving
Cooking Time:
20 minutes (assuming rice and beans are pre-cooked)

Instructions:

1. In a bowl, layer cooked brown rice, black beans, grilled chicken, shredded lettuce, tomato salsa, guacamole, Greek yogurt or sour cream, and shredded cheese.
2. Mix and enjoy this customizable and PCOS-friendly Zambrero's Burrito Bowl.

Harvest Chicken Chili

Harvest chicken chili provides a combination of protein and fiber from chicken and vegetables, supporting satiety and blood sugar control in PCOS patients.

Ingredients:
- Ground chicken (1 lb)
- Onion (1, diced)
- Bell peppers (2, diced)
- Sweet potatoes (2 cups, diced)
- Black beans (1 can, drained and rinsed)
- Diced tomatoes (1 can)
- Chicken broth (2 cups)
- Chili powder (2 tablespoons)
- Cumin (1 tablespoon)
- Paprika (1 teaspoon)
- Salt and pepper to taste

Serving Size:
6 servings
Cooking Time:
30 minutes

Instructions:

1. In a large pot, cook ground chicken until browned.

2. Add diced onion, bell peppers, and sweet potatoes. Keep cooking until the vegetables become soft.

3. Stir in black beans, diced tomatoes, chicken broth, chili powder, cumin, paprika, salt, and pepper.

4. Simmer for 20 minutes or until the sweet potatoes are tender.

5. Serve and enjoy this hearty Harvest Chicken Chili.

Zuppa Toscana

Zuppa Toscana, with its combination of lean turkey sausage and nutrient-rich kale, provides a hearty and flavorful soup option that supports a balanced diet for PCOS patients.

Ingredients:
- Turkey sausage (1 lb, crumbled)
- Kale (4 cups, chopped)
- Potatoes (2, diced)
- Onion (1, diced)
- Garlic cloves (3, minced)
- Chicken broth (4 cups)
- Heavy cream (1 cup)
- Red pepper flakes (1/2 teaspoon)
- Salt and pepper to taste

Serving Size:
6 servings
Cooking Time:
30 minutes

Instructions:

1. In a large pot, brown the crumbled turkey sausage.
2. Add diced onion and minced garlic. Cook until softened.
3. Stir in diced potatoes, chopped kale, chicken broth, red pepper flakes, salt, and pepper.
4. Simmer until potatoes are cooked through.
5. Pour in heavy cream, heat through, and serve this PCOS-friendly Zuppa Toscana.

Shrimp Fried Rice

Shrimp fried rice offers a low-carb alternative to traditional fried rice, providing lean protein from shrimp and a mix of vegetables for a balanced meal.

Ingredients:
- Shrimp (1 lb, peeled and deveined)
- Brown rice (2 cups, cooked)
- Mixed vegetables (1 cup, diced)
- Eggs (2, beaten)
- Soy sauce (2 tablespoons)
- Sesame oil (1 tablespoon)
- Green onions (2, chopped)
- Garlic powder (1/2 teaspoon)

Serving Size:
4 servings
Cooking Time:
20 minutes

Instructions:
1. In a pan, cook shrimp until pink. Set aside.
2. In the same pan, add mixed vegetables and cook until tender.
3. Push vegetables to the side, add beaten eggs, and scramble.
4. Add cooked brown rice, cooked shrimp, soy sauce, sesame oil, garlic powder, and chopped green onions.
5. Stir well and enjoy this quick and PCOS-friendly Shrimp Fried Rice.

Slow Cooked Beef and Broccoli

Slow-cooked beef and broccoli provide a good source of protein and fiber, supporting satiety and blood sugar control for PCOS patients.

Ingredients:
- Beef chuck roast (2 lbs, thinly sliced)
- Broccoli florets (4 cups)
- Soy sauce (1/2 cup)
- Beef broth (1/2 cup)
- Garlic cloves (3, minced)
- Ginger (1 teaspoon, minced)
- Sesame oil (1 tablespoon)
- Brown sugar or sweetener (2 tablespoons)
- Cornstarch (2 tablespoons, optional for thickening)

Serving Size:
6 servings
Cooking Time:
4-6 hours (slow cooker)

Instructions:

1. In a slow cooker, combine sliced beef, broccoli florets, soy sauce, beef broth, minced garlic, minced ginger, sesame oil, and brown sugar.

2. Cook on low for 4-6 hours.

3. If desired, mix cornstarch with water and stir into the slow cooker to thicken the sauce.

4. Serve and enjoy this flavorful and PCOS-friendly Slow Cooked Beef and Broccoli.

Keto Pizza

Keto pizza provides a low-carb alternative to traditional pizza, offering a satisfying option with healthy fats and protein for PCOS patients.

Ingredients:
- Cauliflower (1 head, riced)
- Mozzarella cheese (2 cups, shredded)
- Eggs (2)
- Tomato sauce (1/2 cup)
- Pepperoni or your preferred toppings
- Olive oil (1 tablespoon)
- Italian seasoning (1 teaspoon)
- Salt and pepper to taste

Serving Size:
4 servings
Cooking Time:
30 minutes

1. Before you start cooking, heat the oven to 425°F (220°C).

2. Combine riced cauliflower, shredded mozzarella cheese, and beaten eggs in a bowl.

3. Press the mixture onto a parchment-lined baking sheet to form a pizza crust.

4. Bake for 20 minutes or until the crust is golden brown.

5. Spread tomato sauce over the crust, add toppings, and drizzle with olive oil.

6. Bake for an additional 10 minutes.

7. Sprinkle with Italian seasoning, salt, and pepper.

8. Slice and enjoy this low-carb Keto Pizza.

Healthy Chicken Nuggets

Healthy chicken nuggets offer a protein-rich alternative to traditional nuggets, incorporating lean chicken and whole-grain coating for a balanced and satisfying meal.

Ingredients:

- Chicken breast (1 lb, cut into bite-sized pieces)
- Whole wheat breadcrumbs (1 cup)
- Parmesan cheese (1/4 cup, grated)
- Italian seasoning (1 teaspoon)
- Garlic powder (1/2 teaspoon)
- Paprika (1/2 teaspoon)
- Salt and pepper to taste
- Eggs (2, beaten)

Serving Size:
4 servings
Cooking Time:
20 minutes

Instructions:

1. Get the oven ready by setting it to 400°F (200°C) before you start cooking.

2. In a bowl, mix whole wheat breadcrumbs, grated Parmesan cheese, Italian seasoning, garlic powder, paprika, salt, and pepper.

3. Dip chicken pieces into beaten eggs and then coat with the breadcrumb mixture.

4. Place the coated chicken on a baking sheet.

5. Bake for 15-18 minutes or until golden brown.

6. Serve these PCOS-friendly Healthy Chicken Nuggets with your favorite dipping sauce.

Vegetable Stew

Vegetable stew provides a hearty and fiber-rich option, incorporating a variety of vegetables that support overall health and digestion for PCOS patients.

Ingredients:

- Carrots (2, sliced)

- Potatoes (2, diced)

- Celery (2 stalks, chopped)

- Onion (1, diced)

- Garlic cloves (3, minced)

- Tomato sauce (1 cup)

- Vegetable broth (4 cups)

- Mixed vegetables (2 cups, e.g., green beans, peas, corn)

- Bay leaves (2)

- Thyme (1 teaspoon, dried)

- Salt and pepper to taste

Serving Size:

6 servings

Cooking Time:

30 minutes

Instructions:

1. In a pot, sauté onions and garlic until fragrant.

2. Add carrots, potatoes, celery, tomato sauce, vegetable broth, mixed vegetables, bay leaves, thyme, salt, and pepper.

3. Bring to a boil, then reduce heat and simmer for 20-25 minutes or until vegetables are tender.

4. Remove bay leaves before serving.

5. Enjoy this comforting and PCOS-friendly Vegetable Stew on its own or with whole grains for added fiber.

Dessert Recipes

Chocolate Mud Cake

This chocolate mud cake offers a satisfying dessert option with reduced sugar and whole-grain flour, making it a better choice for managing blood sugar levels.

Ingredients:
- Whole wheat flour (1 cup)
- Cocoa powder (1/2 cup)
- Baking powder (1 teaspoon)
- Unsweetened applesauce (1/2 cup)
- Greek yogurt (1/2 cup)
- Honey or maple syrup (1/4 cup)
- Eggs (2)
- Vanilla extract (1 teaspoon)
- Dark chocolate chips (1/4 cup)

Serving Size:
8 servings
Cooking Time:
25 minutes

Instructions:

1. Warm up the oven by setting it to 350°F (175°C) before you begin cooking.
2. In a bowl, whisk together whole wheat flour, cocoa powder, and baking powder.
3. In another bowl, mix applesauce, Greek yogurt, honey or maple syrup, eggs, and vanilla extract.
4. Combine wet and dry ingredients until well incorporated.
5. Fold in dark chocolate chips.
6. Pour the batter into a greased cake pan and bake for 20-25 minutes.
7. Allow to cool before slicing and enjoy your Chocolate Mud Cake.

Banana Bread

Banana bread provides a naturally sweet option with ripe bananas and whole-grain flour, offering fiber and nutrients for PCOS patients.

Ingredients:
- Ripe bananas (3, mashed)
- Whole wheat flour (1 1/2 cups)
- Baking soda (1 teaspoon)
- Greek yogurt (1/2 cup)
- Eggs (2)
- Honey or maple syrup (1/2 cup)
- Vanilla extract (1 teaspoon)
- Cinnamon (1 teaspoon)

Serving Size:
10 servings
Cooking Time:
50 minutes

Instructions:

1. Preheat the oven to 350°F (175°C).

2. In a bowl, mash ripe bananas.

3. In another bowl, whisk together whole wheat flour and baking soda.

4. In a separate bowl, mix Greek yogurt, eggs, honey or maple syrup, vanilla extract, and cinnamon.

5. Combine wet and dry ingredients until well blended.

6. Pour the batter into a greased loaf pan and bake for 45-50 minutes.

7. Allow to cool before slicing and enjoy this PCOS-friendly Banana Bread.

Berry Delight

Berry Delight offers a refreshing and antioxidant-rich dessert with a mix of berries, supporting overall health and inflammation reduction in PCOS patients.

Ingredients:
- Mixed berries (2 cups, e.g., strawberries, blueberries, raspberries)
- Greek yogurt (1 cup)
- Honey (2 tablespoons)
- Mint leaves (for garnish)

Serving Size:
2 servings
Cooking Time:
No cooking required

1. In a bowl, mix mixed berries with Greek yogurt.
2. Drizzle honey over the berries and yogurt.
3. Garnish with mint leaves.
4. Serve and enjoy this simple Berry Delight.

Ginger Cookies

Ginger cookies offer a flavorful treat with the potential anti-inflammatory properties of ginger, providing a delicious option.

Ingredients:
- Whole wheat flour (1 cup)
- Almond flour (1/2 cup)
- Baking soda (1/2 teaspoon)
- Ground ginger (1 teaspoon)
- Cinnamon (1/2 teaspoon)
- Coconut oil (1/4 cup, melted)
- Molasses (1/4 cup)
- Maple syrup (1/4 cup)
- Egg (1)
- Vanilla extract (1 teaspoon)

Serving Size:
12 cookies
Cooking Time:
10 minutes

Instructions:

1. Preheat the oven to 350°F (175°C).

2. In a bowl, whisk together whole wheat flour, almond flour, baking soda, ground ginger, and cinnamon.

3. In another bowl, mix melted coconut oil, molasses, maple syrup, egg, and vanilla extract.

4. Combine wet and dry ingredients until a dough forms.

5. Roll dough into balls and place on a baking sheet.

6. Flatten each ball with a fork.

7. Bake for 8-10 minutes.

8. Allow to cool before serving these PCOS-friendly Ginger Cookies.

Chai Tea Frozen Yogurt

Chai tea frozen yogurt offers a lower-sugar alternative to traditional desserts, incorporating the warm flavors of chai tea with the probiotic benefits of yogurt for digestive health in PCOS patients.

Ingredients:
- Greek yogurt (2 cups)
- Chai tea concentrate (1/4 cup)
- Honey or maple syrup (2 tablespoons)
- Vanilla extract (1 teaspoon)
- Ground cinnamon (1/2 teaspoon)
- Ground cardamom (1/4 teaspoon)

Serving Size:
4 servings
Cooking Time:
4 hours (freezing time)

Instructions:

1. In a bowl, whisk together Greek yogurt, chai tea concentrate, honey or maple syrup, vanilla extract, ground cinnamon, and ground cardamom.

2. Pour the mixture into a freezer-safe container.

3. Freeze for at least 4 hours before serving.

4. Remove the frozen yogurt from the freezer and let it sit at room temperature for a few minutes to soften slightly.

5. Scoop the Chai Tea Frozen Yogurt into bowls or cones.

6. Garnish with a sprinkle of additional cinnamon or a drizzle of honey if desired.

7. Enjoy this delightful Chai Tea Frozen Yogurt.

Snacks Recipes

Trail Mix

Trail mix offers a balanced combination of nuts, seeds, and dried fruits, providing healthy fats, protein, and fiber to support satiety and stable blood sugar levels in PCOS patients.

Ingredients:

- Almonds (1/2 cup)

- Walnuts (1/2 cup)

- Pumpkin seeds (1/4 cup)

- Dried cranberries (1/4 cup)

- Dark chocolate chips (1/4 cup)

Serving Size:

4 servings

Cooking Time:

No cooking required

Instructions:

1. In a bowl, mix almonds, walnuts, pumpkin seeds, dried cranberries, and dark chocolate chips.

2. Portion the trail mix into individual servings.

3. Enjoy this PCOS-friendly Trail Mix as a satisfying and nutrient-packed snack.

Guacamole

Guacamole provides a delicious and nutrient-dense snack with avocados, offering healthy monounsaturated fats and various vitamins and minerals.

Ingredients:

- Avocados (2, mashed)
- Tomato (1, diced)
- Red onion (1/4 cup, finely chopped)
- Fresh cilantro (2 tablespoons, chopped)
- Lime juice (1-2 tablespoons)
- Salt and pepper to taste

Serving Size:
4 servings
Cooking Time:
No cooking required

Instructions:

1. Take a bowl and use a fork to crush the avocados inside.

2. Add diced tomato, finely chopped red onion, chopped fresh cilantro, lime juice, salt, and pepper.

3. Mix well until ingredients are combined.

4. Serve this Guacamole with whole-grain chips or vegetable sticks for dipping.

Zucchini Chips

Zucchini chips provide a crunchy and low-carb snack option, offering a satisfying alternative to traditional potato chips while contributing to a balanced diet for PCOS patients.

Ingredients:

- Zucchini (2, thinly sliced)

- Olive oil (1 tablespoon)

- Parmesan cheese (2 tablespoons, grated)

- Garlic powder (1/2 teaspoon)

- Paprika (1/2 teaspoon)

- Salt and pepper to taste

Serving Size:

2 servings

Cooking Time:

25 minutes

Instructions:

1. Before you start cooking, heat the oven to 400°F (200°C).

2. In a bowl, toss thinly sliced zucchini with olive oil, grated Parmesan cheese, garlic powder, paprika, salt, and pepper.

3. Arrange the zucchini slices on a baking sheet in a single layer.

4. Bake for 20-25 minutes or until the chips are golden and crisp.

5. Allow to cool before serving these PCOS-friendly Zucchini Chips as a tasty and guilt-free snack.

Beef Jerky

Beef jerky is a portable and protein-rich snack, providing satiety and supporting muscle health for PCOS patients. It's a convenient option for on-the-go energy.

Ingredients:

- Lean beef (1 lb, thinly sliced)
- Soy sauce (1/4 cup)
- Worcestershire sauce (2 tablespoons)
- Honey or maple syrup (1 tablespoon)
- Garlic powder (1 teaspoon)
- Onion powder (1 teaspoon)
- Black pepper (1/2 teaspoon)

Serving Size:

4 servings

Cooking Time:

4-6 hours (dehydrator) or 2-3 hours (oven)

1. In a bowl, mix soy sauce, Worcestershire sauce, honey or maple syrup, garlic powder, onion powder, and black pepper.

2. Place thinly sliced beef in the marinade, ensuring each piece is coated.

3. Marinate for at least 2 hours or overnight in the refrigerator.

4. If using a dehydrator, follow the manufacturer's instructions. If using an oven, preheat to the lowest setting (usually around 170°F or 75°C) and place the beef on a rack over a baking sheet.

5. Dehydrate for 4-6 hours in a dehydrator 2-3 hours in an oven, or until the beef is dried and chewy.

6. Allow to cool before enjoying this Beef Jerky.

Apple (or Any Fruit) or Celery and Nut Butter

This snack provides a combination of fiber from the fruit or celery and healthy fats from nut butter, offering a balanced and satisfying option for PCOS patients.

Ingredients:

- Apples or any fruit of choice (2, sliced) OR Celery sticks (4-6)
- Nut butter (almond, peanut, or any preferred, 4 tablespoons)

Serving Size:
2 servings
Cooking Time:
No cooking required

1. Slice apples or any preferred fruit or prepare celery sticks.

2. Pair the fruit or celery with nut butter for dipping.

3. Enjoy this quick and PCOS-friendly Apple (or Any Fruit) or Celery + Nut Butter snack for a delightful combination of sweetness and crunch.

Smoothies Recipes

Supercharged Green Smoothie

The Supercharged Green Smoothie offers a nutrient-packed blend of leafy greens and fruits, providing essential vitamins and minerals, along with fiber for improved digestion and hormonal balance.

Ingredients:

- Spinach (2 cups, fresh)

- Kale (1 cup, fresh)

- Banana (1, frozen)

- Pineapple chunks (1/2 cup, frozen)

- Greek yogurt (1/2 cup)

- Chia seeds (1 tablespoon)

- Almond milk (1 cup)

- Ice cubes (1/2 cup)

Serving Size:

2 servings

Preparation Time:

5 minutes

Instructions:

1. In a blender, combine spinach, kale, frozen banana, frozen pineapple chunks, Greek yogurt, chia seeds, almond milk, and ice cubes.

2. Mix everything until it becomes smooth and creamy.

3. Pour into glasses and enjoy this refreshing and PCOS-friendly Supercharged Green Smoothie.

Nutty Chai Smoothie

The Nutty Chai Smoothie combines the warmth of chai spices with the richness of nuts, offering a flavorful and satisfying smoothie with protein and healthy fats.

Ingredients:
- Chai tea concentrate (1/2 cup, cooled)
- Almond butter (2 tablespoons)
- Banana (1, frozen)
- Greek yogurt (1/2 cup)
- Almond milk (1 cup)
- Ice cubes (1/2 cup)
- Cinnamon (1/2 teaspoon)

Serving Size:
2 servings
Preparation Time:
5 minutes

Instructions:

1. Brew chai tea and let it cool.

2. In a blender, combine chai tea concentrate, almond butter, frozen banana, Greek yogurt, almond milk, ice cubes, and cinnamon.

3. Mix everything until it becomes smooth and creamy.

4. Pour into glasses and savor the delicious and PCOS-friendly Nutty Chai Smoothie.

Spicy Veggie Smoothie

The Spicy Veggie Smoothie provides a unique twist with a kick of spice, incorporating vegetables for added nutrients and a metabolism boost, supporting weight management in PCOS patients.

Ingredients:
- Tomato (1, diced)
- Cucumber (1/2, peeled and sliced)
- Celery (2 stalks, chopped)
- Jalapeño (1/2, seeded and chopped)
- Lemon juice (2 tablespoons)
- Greek yogurt (1/2 cup)
- Ice cubes (1/2 cup)
- Water (1/2 cup)
- Salt and black pepper to taste

Serving Size:

2 servings

Preparation Time:

5 minutes

Instructions:

1. In a blender, combine diced tomato, sliced cucumber, chopped celery, chopped jalapeño, lemon juice, Greek yogurt, ice cubes, water, salt, and black pepper.

2. Blend until smooth and slightly spicy.

3. Pour into glasses and enjoy this invigorating and PCOS-friendly Spicy Veggie Smoothie.

Chocolate Chia Pudding

Chocolate Chia Pudding is a rich and satisfying dessert that provides a dose of healthy fats, fiber, and antioxidants. Chia seeds are a good source of omega-3 fatty acids and can contribute to improved blood sugar control.

Ingredients:

- Chia seeds (1/4 cup)

- Unsweetened cocoa powder (2 tablespoons)

- Greek yogurt (1/2 cup)

- Almond milk (1 cup)

- Use one teaspoon of vanilla extract.

- Maple syrup or honey (2 tablespoons)

Serving Size:

2 servings

Preparation Time:

5 minutes (plus chilling time)

1. In a bowl, mix chia seeds, cocoa powder, Greek yogurt, almond milk, vanilla extract, and maple syrup or honey.

2. Stir well to combine and ensure that chia seeds are evenly distributed.

3. Refrigerate for at least 4 hours or overnight to allow the pudding to thicken.

4. Before serving, give it a good stir, and enjoy this Chocolate Chia Pudding.

Chai Tea Frozen Yogurt

Chai Tea Frozen Yogurt offers a delightful frozen treat with the warm and comforting flavors of chai tea. Greek yogurt provides probiotics for gut health, and the controlled sweetness makes it a better dessert option for PCOS patients.

Ingredients:

- Greek yogurt (2 cups)

- Chai tea concentrate (1/4 cup)

- Honey or maple syrup (2 tablespoons)

- Vanilla extract (1 teaspoon)

- Add half a teaspoon of ground cinnamon.

- Ground cardamom (1/4 teaspoon)

Serving Size:

4 servings

Preparation Time:

4 hours (freezing time)

1. In a bowl, whisk together Greek yogurt, chai tea concentrate, honey or maple syrup, vanilla extract, ground cinnamon, and ground cardamom.

2. Pour the mixture into a freezer-safe container.

3. Freeze for at least 4 hours before serving this delicious Chai Tea Frozen Yogurt.

Fertility Smoothie Avocado Berry

The Avocado Berry Fertility Smoothie is designed to incorporate nutrient-rich ingredients, such as avocado and berries, which are high in antioxidants and healthy fats. This combination may support hormonal balance and overall fertility.

Ingredients:

- Avocado (1/2, peeled and pitted)
- Mixed berries (1 cup, e.g., strawberries, blueberries, raspberries)
- Greek yogurt (1/2 cup)
- Flaxseeds (1 tablespoon)
- Honey or agave syrup (1 tablespoon)
- Almond milk (1 cup)

Serving Size:
2 servings
Preparation Time:
5 minutes

Instructions:

1. In a blender, combine avocado, mixed berries, Greek yogurt, flaxseeds, honey or agave syrup, and almond milk.

2. Mix everything all together until it turns smooth and creamy.

3. Pour into glasses and enjoy this nutrient-packed and PCOS-friendly Avocado Berry Fertility Smoothie.

Creamy Mango Pineapple Smoothie

The Creamy Mango Pineapple Smoothie is a tropical delight that offers a sweet and refreshing option while providing essential vitamins and minerals. The combination of mango and pineapple adds a burst of flavor and antioxidants.

Ingredients:
- Mango (1 cup, frozen)
- Pineapple chunks (1/2 cup, frozen)
- Greek yogurt (1/2 cup)
- Almond milk (1 cup)
- Chia seeds (1 tablespoon)
- Honey or agave syrup (1 tablespoon)
Serving Size:
2 servings
Preparation Time:
5 minutes

Instructions:

1. In a blender, combine frozen mango, frozen pineapple chunks, Greek yogurt, almond milk, chia seeds, and honey or agave syrup.

2. Blend until smooth and creamy.

3. Pour into glasses and enjoy this tropical Creamy Mango Pineapple Smoothie.

Low Carb Green Smoothie

The Low Carb Green Smoothie is a nutrient-dense option that focuses on low-carb vegetables and healthy fats, making it suitable for PCOS patients aiming for balanced blood sugar levels.

Ingredients:
- Spinach (2 cups, fresh)
- Avocado (1/2, peeled and pitted)
- Cucumber (1/2, peeled)
- Coconut milk (1/2 cup)
- Water (1/2 cup)
- Lime juice (1-2 tablespoons)
- Stevia or your preferred low-carb sweetener (to taste)
- Ice cubes (1/2 cup)

Serving Size:
2 servings
Preparation Time:
5 minutes

Instructions:

1. In a blender, combine fresh spinach, avocado, peeled cucumber, coconut milk, water, lime juice, stevia, and ice cubes.

2. Blend until smooth.

3. Pour into glasses and enjoy this nutrient-packed and PCOS-friendly Carb Green Smoothie.

Iced Coffee Protein Shake

The Iced Coffee Protein Shake provides a satisfying and energizing drink with the benefits of protein. It's a great way to incorporate protein into the diet, supporting muscle health and satiety for PCOS patients.

Ingredients:
- Cold brew coffee (1 cup)
- Protein powder (vanilla or chocolate, 2 scoops)
- Almond milk (1/2 cup)
- Ice cubes (1/2 cup)
- Stevia or your preferred sweetener (to taste)

Serving Size:
2 servings
Preparation Time:
5 minutes

Instructions:
1. In a blender, combine cold brew coffee, protein powder, almond milk, ice cubes, and sweetener.
2. Blend until smooth and frothy.
3. Pour into glasses and enjoy this refreshing and PCOS-friendly Iced Coffee Protein Shake.

Strawberry Banana Peanut Butter Smoothie

The Strawberry Banana Peanut Butter Smoothie combines the sweetness of fruits with the richness of peanut butter, offering a tasty and protein-packed option that supports energy and satiety for PCOS patients.

Ingredients:
- Strawberries (1 cup, frozen)
- Banana (1, frozen)
- Peanut butter (2 tablespoons)
- Greek yogurt (1/2 cup)
- Almond milk (1 cup)

Serving Size:
2 servings
Preparation Time:
5 minutes

Instructions:

1. In a blender, combine frozen strawberries, frozen banana, peanut butter, Greek yogurt, and almond milk.

2. Mix everything all together until it turns creamy and smooth.

3. Pour into glasses and enjoy this delicious and PCOS-friendly Strawberry Banana Peanut Butter Smoothie.

Soup Recipes

Apple and Onion Soup

Apple and Onion Soup provides a unique blend of flavors and incorporates apples, which may contribute to improved insulin sensitivity. The fiber content supports digestive health for PCOS patients.

Ingredients:

- Onions (2 large, thinly sliced)
- Apples (2, peeled and sliced)
- Vegetable broth (4 cups)
- Olive oil (2 tablespoons)
- Thyme (1 teaspoon, dried)
- Bay leaves (2)
- Salt and pepper to taste

Serving Size:
4 servings
Cooking Time:
40 minutes

1. In a pot, heat olive oil over medium heat. Add thinly sliced onions and cook until caramelized.

2. Add sliced apples, thyme, bay leaves, salt, and pepper. Cook for an additional 5 minutes.

3. Put the vegetable broth in the pot and let it boil. Then, lower the heat and let it simmer for 30 minutes.

4. Remove bay leaves and blend the soup until smooth.

5. Serve this Apple and Onion Soup warm, garnished with fresh thyme if desired.

Super-Healthy Gazpacho Soup

Super-Healthy Gazpacho Soup is packed with vegetables, providing a low-calorie and nutrient-dense option. The inclusion of tomatoes and cucumbers may contribute to antioxidant intake.

Ingredients:

- Tomatoes (4, diced)

- Cucumber (1, peeled and diced)

- Bell pepper (1, diced)

- Red onion (1/2, diced)

- Garlic cloves (2, minced)

- Tomato juice (2 cups)

- Olive oil (2 tablespoons)

- Red wine vinegar (2 tablespoons)

- Basil (1/4 cup, fresh, chopped)

- Salt and pepper to taste

Serving Size:

4 servings

Preparation Time:

15 minutes

Instructions:

1. In a blender, combine diced tomatoes, diced cucumber, diced bell pepper, minced garlic, tomato juice, olive oil, red wine vinegar, fresh basil, salt, and pepper.

2. Blend until smooth.

3. Chill the soup in the refrigerator for at least 2 hours.

4. Serve this PCOS-friendly Super-Healthy Gazpacho Soup cold, garnished with additional fresh basil.

Tangy Tomato Soup with Basil

Tangy Tomato Soup with Basil offers a classic and flavorful option with tomatoes that contain antioxidants, including lycopene. Basil adds a refreshing touch and potential anti-inflammatory properties.

Ingredients:
- Tomatoes (6, diced)
- Onion (1, diced)
- Garlic cloves (3, minced)
- Vegetable broth (4 cups)
- Olive oil (2 tablespoons)
- Tomato paste (2 tablespoons)
- Fresh basil (1/4 cup, chopped)
- Salt and pepper to taste

Serving Size:
4 servings
Cooking Time:
30 minutes

Instructions:

1. In a pot, warm up olive oil on medium heat. Put in chopped onions and cook until they become soft.

2. Include minced garlic and cook for one more minute.

3. Stir in diced tomatoes, tomato paste, vegetable broth, salt, and pepper. Simmer for 20 minutes.

4. Blend the soup until smooth. Stir in fresh basil.

5. Serve this Tangy Tomato Soup with Basil hot, garnished with additional basil if desired.

Wholesome Winter Pea and Watercress Soup

Wholesome Winter Pea and Watercress Soup brings together the goodness of peas and watercress. Peas offer plant-based protein and fiber, while watercress adds a dose of vitamins and minerals, promoting overall health for PCOS patients.

Ingredients:

- Peas (2 cups, frozen)

- Watercress (1 bunch, stems removed)

- Onion (1, diced)

- Vegetable broth (4 cups)

- Olive oil (2 tablespoons)

- Garlic cloves (2, minced)

- Mint leaves (1/4 cup, fresh, chopped)

- Salt and pepper to taste

Serving Size:

4 servings

Cooking Time:

30 minutes

1. In a pot, heat olive oil over medium heat. Add diced onion and cook until softened.

2. Add minced garlic and cook for an additional minute.

3. Stir in frozen peas, watercress, vegetable broth, salt, and pepper. Simmer for 20 minutes.

4. Blend the soup until smooth. Stir in fresh mint.

5. Serve this Wholesome Winter Pea and Watercress Soup hot, garnished with additional mint if desired.

Carrot, Tomato, and Lentil Soup

Carrot, Tomato, and Lentil Soup provide a nutrient-rich combination with carrots offering beta-carotene, tomatoes contributing antioxidants, and lentils providing protein and fiber for improved satiety.

Ingredients:

- Carrots (3, peeled and sliced)
- Tomatoes (4, diced)
- Red lentils (1 cup)
- Onion (1, diced)
- Garlic cloves (3, minced)
- Vegetable broth (4 cups)
- Olive oil (2 tablespoons)
- Cumin (1 teaspoon, ground)
- Paprika (1 teaspoon)
- Salt and pepper to taste

Serving Size:

4 servings

Cooking Time:

40 minutes

Instructions:

1. In a pot, heat olive oil over medium heat. Add diced onion and cook until softened.

2. Add minced garlic, ground cumin, and paprika. Cook for an additional minute.

3. Stir in sliced carrots, diced tomatoes, red lentils, vegetable broth, salt, and pepper. Simmer for 30 minutes.

4. Blend the soup until smooth.

5. Serve this PCOS-friendly Carrot, Tomato, and Lentil Soup hot, garnished with a drizzle of olive oil if desired.

Iced Watercress and Mint Soup

Iced Watercress and Mint Soup offer a refreshing option with watercress providing vitamins and minerals. The cooling nature of this soup can be soothing, making it a pleasant choice for PCOS patients.

Ingredients:

- Watercress (1 bunch, stems removed)

- Fresh mint (1/2 cup, chopped)

- Cucumber (1, peeled and chopped)

- Greek yogurt (1 cup)

- Vegetable broth (1 cup)

- Lemon juice (2 tablespoons)

- Salt and pepper to taste

Serving Size:

4 servings

Preparation Time:

10 minutes (plus chilling time)

Instructions:

1. In a blender, combine watercress, fresh mint, chopped cucumber, Greek yogurt, vegetable broth, lemon juice, salt, and pepper.

2. Blend until smooth.

3. Chill the soup in the refrigerator for at least 2 hours.

4. Serve this Iced Watercress and Mint Soup cold, garnished with additional mint if desired.

Creamy Broccoli Soup

Creamy Broccoli Soup provides a good source of fiber and nutrients from broccoli. The inclusion of dairy-free alternatives makes it suitable for those with lactose sensitivities often associated with PCOS.

Ingredients:
- Broccoli (2 cups, chopped)
- Onion (1, diced)
- Vegetable broth (4 cups)
- Coconut milk (1 cup)
- Nutritional yeast (2 tablespoons)
- Olive oil (2 tablespoons)
- Garlic cloves (2, minced)
- Salt and pepper to taste

Serving Size:
4 servings
Cooking Time:
30 minutes

Instructions:

1. In a pot, heat olive oil over medium heat. Add diced onion and cook until softened.

2. Add minced garlic and cook for an additional minute.

3. Stir in chopped broccoli, vegetable broth, coconut milk, nutritional yeast, salt, and pepper. Simmer for 20 minutes.

4. Blend the soup until smooth.

5. Serve this PCOS-friendly Creamy Broccoli Soup hot, garnished with a drizzle of coconut milk if desired.

Slow Cooker Chicken Soup

Slow Cooker Chicken Soup offers a convenient and comforting option with chicken providing lean protein. The slow cooking process allows flavors to meld, creating a wholesome dish for PCOS patients.

Ingredients:
- Chicken breasts (2, boneless and skinless)
- Carrots (3, peeled and sliced)
- Celery (3 stalks, chopped)
- Onion (1, diced)
- Garlic cloves (3, minced)
- Chicken broth (6 cups)
- Thyme (1 teaspoon, dried)
- Bay leaves (2)
- Salt and pepper to taste

Serving Size:
6 servings
Cooking Time:
4-6 hours (slow cooker)

Instructions:

1. Place chicken breasts, sliced carrots, chopped celery, diced onion, minced garlic, chicken broth, thyme, bay leaves, salt, and pepper in a slow cooker.

2. Cook on low for 4-6 hours or until chicken is cooked through.

3. Shred the chicken and return it to the slow cooker.

4. Serve this PCOS-friendly Slow Cooker Chicken Soup hot, garnished with fresh herbs if desired.

Spicy Pumpkin Soup

Spicy Pumpkin Soup combines the nutritional benefits of pumpkin with warming spices. Pumpkin is rich in vitamins and antioxidants, potentially supporting immune health for PCOS patients.

Ingredients:
- Pumpkin puree (2 cups)
- Onion (1, diced)
- Vegetable broth (4 cups)
- Coconut milk (1/2 cup)
- Curry powder (1 teaspoon)
- Ground cinnamon (1/2 teaspoon)
- Cayenne pepper (1/4 teaspoon, optional)
- Olive oil (2 tablespoons)
- Salt and pepper to taste

Serving Size:
4 servings
Cooking Time:
25 minutes

1. In a pot, warm olive oil on medium heat. Put in chopped onions and cook until they become soft.

2. Add pumpkin puree, vegetable broth, coconut milk, curry powder, ground cinnamon, cayenne pepper (if using), salt, and pepper. Simmer for 15 minutes.

3. Blend the soup until smooth.

4. Serve this PCOS-friendly Spicy Pumpkin Soup hot, garnished with a swirl of coconut milk if desired.

Creamy Cauliflower Soup

Creamy Cauliflower Soup offers a low-carb alternative with cauliflower as the base. Cauliflower is rich in fiber and antioxidants, contributing to a balanced diet for PCOS patients.

Ingredients:
- Cauliflower (1 head, chopped)
- Onion (1, diced)
- Garlic cloves (3, minced)
- Vegetable broth (4 cups)
- Coconut milk (1/2 cup)
- Nutritional yeast (2 tablespoons)
- Olive oil (2 tablespoons)
- Thyme (1 teaspoon, dried)
- Salt and pepper to taste

Serving Size:
4 servings
Cooking Time:
30 minutes

Instructions:

1. In a pot, heat olive oil over medium heat. Add diced onion and cook until softened.

2. Include minced garlic and continue cooking for one more minute.

3. Stir in chopped cauliflower, vegetable broth, coconut milk, nutritional yeast, thyme, salt, and pepper. Simmer for 20 minutes.

4. Blend the soup until smooth.

5. Serve this PCOS-friendly Creamy Cauliflower Soup hot, garnished with a sprinkle of thyme if desired.

Salad Recipes

Tomato, Cucumber, and Red Onion Salad

Tomato, Cucumber, and Red Onion Salad offer a light and refreshing option with tomatoes providing antioxidants, cucumbers contributing hydration, and red onions potentially supporting anti-inflammatory properties.

Ingredients:

- Tomatoes (2 cups, cherry or grape tomatoes, halved)
- Cucumber (1, thinly sliced)
- Red onion (1/2, thinly sliced)
- Olive oil (2 tablespoons)
- Balsamic vinegar (1 tablespoon)
- Fresh basil (1/4 cup, chopped)
- Salt and pepper to taste

Serving Size:

4 servings

Preparation Time:

10 minutes

Instructions:

1. In a bowl, combine halved cherry or grape tomatoes, thinly sliced cucumber, and thinly sliced red onion.

2. Drizzle olive oil and balsamic vinegar over the salad.

3. Add chopped fresh basil, salt, and pepper. Toss gently to combine.

4. Serve this PCOS-friendly Tomato, Cucumber, and Red Onion Salad chilled.

Super-Nutritious Broccoli Salad with Apples and Cranberries

Super-Nutritious Broccoli Salad with Apples and Cranberries combines nutrient-dense broccoli with the natural sweetness of apples and cranberries. This salad offers fiber and antioxidants beneficial for PCOS patients.

Ingredients:

- Broccoli florets (4 cups, chopped)
- Apples (2, diced)
- Dried cranberries (1/2 cup)
- Red onion (1/4 cup, finely chopped)
- Sunflower seeds (1/4 cup)
- Greek yogurt (1/2 cup)
- Honey (2 tablespoons)
- Apple cider vinegar (2 tablespoons)
- Salt and pepper to taste

Serving Size:

4 servings

Preparation Time:

15 minutes

Instructions:

1. In a bowl, combine chopped broccoli florets, diced apples, dried cranberries, finely chopped red onion, and sunflower seeds.

2. In a separate small bowl, mix Greek yogurt, honey, apple cider vinegar, salt, and pepper.

3. Pour the dressing over the salad and toss to coat evenly.

4. Serve this Super-Nutritious Broccoli Salad with Apples and Cranberries chilled.

Salmon Salad

Salmon Salad provides a protein-rich option with omega-3 fatty acids from salmon, promoting heart health and potentially offering anti-inflammatory benefits.

Ingredients:

- Salmon fillets (2, cooked and flaked)
- Take four cups of mixed salad greens.
- Cherry tomatoes (1 cup, halved)
- Cucumber (1, sliced)
- Red onion (1/4 cup, thinly sliced)
- Avocado (1, diced)
- Olive oil (2 tablespoons)
- Lemon juice (2 tablespoons)
- Dijon mustard (1 teaspoon)
- Salt and pepper to taste

Serving Size:

2 servings

Preparation Time:

15 minutes

1. In a large bowl, combine cooked and flaked salmon, mixed salad greens, halved cherry tomatoes, sliced cucumber, thinly sliced red onion, and diced avocado.

2. In a small bowl, whisk together olive oil, lemon juice, Dijon mustard, salt, and pepper.

3. Drizzle the dressing over the salad and toss gently to combine.

4. Serve this Salmon Salad immediately, garnished with additional lemon slices if desired.

Beet and Goat Cheese Salad

Beet and Goat Cheese Salad combines the earthy flavors of beets with the creamy richness of goat cheese. Beets may contribute to improved blood flow, while goat cheese provides a source of protein and healthy fats for PCOS patients.

Ingredients:

- Beets (3, roasted and sliced)

- Mixed salad greens (4 cups)

- Goat cheese (1/2 cup, crumbled)

- Walnuts (1/4 cup, chopped)

- Balsamic vinegar (2 tablespoons)

- Olive oil (2 tablespoons)

- Honey (1 tablespoon)

- Salt and pepper to taste

Serving Size:

2 servings

Preparation Time:

20 minutes (including roasting time for beets)

Instructions:

1. Roast beets until tender, peel, and slice.

2. In a bowl, combine mixed salad greens, roasted and sliced beets, crumbled goat cheese, and chopped walnuts.

3. In a small bowl, whisk together balsamic vinegar, olive oil, honey, salt, and pepper.

4. Drizzle the dressing over the salad and toss gently to combine.

5. Serve this Beet and Goat Cheese Salad immediately.

Guacamole Chicken Salad

Guacamole Chicken Salad provides a protein-packed salad with the richness of avocados. Avocados offer healthy fats and may contribute to improved insulin sensitivity for PCOS patients.

Ingredients:
- Chicken breasts (2, cooked and diced)
- Romaine lettuce (4 cups, chopped)
- Cherry tomatoes (1 cup, halved)
- Avocado (2, diced)
- Red onion (1/4 cup, finely chopped)
- Cilantro (1/4 cup, chopped)
- Lime juice (2 tablespoons)
- Olive oil (2 tablespoons)
- Salt and pepper to taste

Serving Size:
2 servings
Preparation Time:
15 minutes

Instructions:

1. In a large bowl, combine cooked and diced chicken breasts, chopped romaine lettuce, halved cherry tomatoes, diced avocado, finely chopped red onion, and chopped cilantro.

2. In a small bowl, whisk together lime juice, olive oil, salt, and pepper.

3. Drizzle the dressing over the salad and toss gently to combine.

4. Serve this PCOS-friendly Guacamole Chicken Salad immediately.

Asian Chicken Slaw

Asian Chicken Slaw offers a crunchy and flavorful salad with cabbage providing fiber and chicken offering lean protein. The variety of vegetables contributes to a nutrient-rich option for PCOS patients.

Ingredients:

- Chicken breasts (2, cooked and shredded)
- Napa cabbage (4 cups, thinly sliced)
- Carrots (2, julienned)
- Red bell pepper (1, thinly sliced)
- Edamame (1/2 cup, cooked)
- Green onions (1/4 cup, sliced)
- Sesame seeds (2 tablespoons)
- Soy sauce (2 tablespoons)
- Rice vinegar (1 tablespoon)
- Sesame oil (1 tablespoon)
- Honey (1 tablespoon)
- Ginger (1 teaspoon, grated)

Serving Size:

4 servings

Preparation Time:

20 minutes

Instructions:

1. In a large bowl, combine cooked and shredded chicken breasts, thinly sliced Napa cabbage, julienned carrots, thinly sliced red bell pepper, cooked edamame, sliced green onions, and sesame seeds.

2. In a small bowl, whisk together soy sauce, rice vinegar, sesame oil, honey, and grated ginger.

3. Drizzle the dressing over the salad and toss gently to combine.

4. Serve this PCOS-friendly Asian Chicken Slaw immediately.

Spinach Chicken Poppers

Spinach Chicken Poppers offer a protein-rich and low-carb option with the added benefits of spinach. Spinach provides iron and other essential nutrients that support overall health, including potential benefits for PCOS patients.

Ingredients:
- Use one pound of ground chicken.
- Spinach (1 cup, cooked and chopped)
- Garlic powder (1 teaspoon)
- Onion powder (1 teaspoon)
- Paprika (1/2 teaspoon)
- Salt and pepper to taste
- Olive oil (1 tablespoon, for cooking)

Serving Size:
4 servings
Cooking Time:
20 minutes

1. In a bowl, combine ground chicken, cooked and chopped spinach, garlic powder, onion powder, paprika, salt, and pepper.

2. Mix the ingredients until well combined.

3. Form the mixture into small poppers or nuggets.

4. Warm up olive oil in a pan on medium heat.

5. Cook the poppers for about 4-5 minutes per side or until fully cooked.

6. Serve these PCOS-friendly Spinach Chicken Poppers hot.

Chicken Collard Wraps

Chicken Collard Wraps offer a low-carb alternative to traditional wraps, providing lean protein from chicken and nutrient-packed collard greens. This recipe supports a balanced and PCOS-friendly diet.

Ingredients:
- Chicken breasts (2, cooked and sliced)
- Collard green leaves (8 large leaves)
- Hummus (1/2 cup)
- Cherry tomatoes (1 cup, halved)
- Cucumber (1, julienned)
- Avocado (1, sliced)
- Red onion (1/4 cup, thinly sliced)

Serving Size:
4 servings
Preparation Time:
15 minutes

Instructions:

1. Blanch collard green leaves in hot water for 30 seconds, then pat them dry.
2. Spread hummus on each collard green leaf.
3. Layer sliced chicken, halved cherry tomatoes, julienned cucumber, avocado slices, and thinly sliced red onion.
4. Roll the collard leaves into wraps.
5. Serve these PCOS-friendly Chicken Collard Wraps immediately.

Sweet Potato Noodle Salad

Sweet Potato Noodle Salad offers a gluten-free alternative with sweet potatoes as the base. Sweet potatoes provide complex carbohydrates and fiber, supporting blood sugar control.

Ingredients:
- Sweet potatoes (2, spiralized or julienned)
- Baby spinach (2 cups)
- Pomegranate seeds (1/2 cup)
- Walnuts (1/4 cup, chopped)
- Feta cheese (1/4 cup, crumbled)
- Olive oil (2 tablespoons)
- Balsamic vinegar (1 tablespoon)
- Salt and pepper to taste

Serving Size:
4 servings
Preparation Time:
20 minutes

1. Spiralize or julienne sweet potatoes.
2. In a bowl, combine sweet potato noodles, baby spinach, pomegranate seeds, chopped walnuts, and crumbled feta cheese.
3. In a small bowl, whisk together olive oil, balsamic vinegar, salt, and pepper.
4. Drizzle the dressing over the salad and toss gently to combine.
5. Serve this Sweet Potato Noodle Salad chilled.

Quinoa Salad with Roasted Vegetables

Quinoa Salad with Roasted Vegetables offers a nutrient-dense option with quinoa providing protein and fiber. The roasted vegetables contribute vitamins and minerals, supporting a well-rounded diet for PCOS patients.

Ingredients:

- Quinoa (1 cup, cooked)
- Bell peppers (2, diced)
- Zucchini (1, diced)
- Cherry tomatoes (1 cup, halved)
- Red onion (1/2, diced)
- Olive oil (2 tablespoons)
- Balsamic vinegar (1 tablespoon)
- Fresh basil (1/4 cup, chopped)
- Salt and pepper to taste

Serving Size:
4 servings
Cooking Time:
25 minutes

Instructions:

1. Cook quinoa according to package instructions.

2. In a bowl, combine cooked quinoa, diced bell peppers, diced zucchini, halved cherry tomatoes, and diced red onion.

3. In a small bowl, whisk together olive oil, balsamic vinegar, chopped fresh basil, salt, and pepper.

4. Drizzle the dressing over the salad and toss gently to combine.

5. Serve this PCOS-friendly Quinoa Salad with Roasted Vegetables chilled or at room temperature.

Side Dish Recipes

Roasted Cauliflower with Pancetta, Olives, & Parmesan

Roasted Cauliflower with Pancetta, Olives, & Parmesan offers a flavorful and low-carb side dish. Cauliflower provides fiber and is a good source of vitamins and minerals, making it a suitable choice for PCOS patients.

Ingredients:

- Cauliflower (1 head, cut into florets)
- Pancetta (1/4 cup, diced)
- Olives (1/4 cup, sliced)
- Parmesan cheese (1/4 cup, grated)
- Olive oil (2 tablespoons)
- Salt and pepper to taste

Serving Size:

4 servings

Cooking Time:

25 minutes

Instructions:

1. Get the oven ready by setting it to 425°F (220°C) before you start cooking.

2. In a large bowl, toss cauliflower florets with diced pancetta, sliced olives, and olive oil.

3. Spread the mixture on a baking sheet and season with salt and pepper.

4. Roast for 20-25 minutes or until cauliflower is golden and tender.

5. Sprinkle-grated Parmesan over the roasted cauliflower before serving.

6. Serve this delicious Roasted Cauliflower with Pancetta, Olives, and parmesan hot.

Zucchini Parmesan

Zucchini Parmesan offers a lighter alternative to traditional eggplant Parmesan. Zucchini is low in carbs and provides essential nutrients, making it a suitable choice for PCOS patients.

Ingredients:

- Zucchini (3, sliced)

- Marinara sauce (1 cup)

- Mozzarella cheese (1 cup, shredded)

- Parmesan cheese (1/2 cup, grated)

- Olive oil (2 tablespoons)

- Italian seasoning (1 teaspoon)

- Salt and pepper to taste

Serving Size:
4 servings
Cooking Time:
30 minutes

1. Warm up the oven by setting it to 375°F (190°C) before you start cooking.

2. In a baking dish, layer sliced zucchini, marinara sauce, mozzarella cheese, and Parmesan cheese.

3. Drizzle with olive oil and sprinkle with Italian seasoning, salt, and pepper.

4. Repeat the layers and finish with a layer of cheese on top.

5. Put it in the oven and let it bake for 25-30 minutes, or until the cheese is melted and bubbly.

6. Serve this PCOS-friendly Zucchini Parmesan hot.

Apple Slaw

Apple Slaw offers a refreshing and nutrient-packed side dish. Apples provide fiber and antioxidants, contributing to a balanced diet for PCOS patients.

Ingredients:

- Apples (2, julienned)
- Cabbage (2 cups, shredded)
- Carrots (1 cup, shredded)
- Greek yogurt (1/2 cup)
- Honey (2 tablespoons)
- Lemon juice (2 tablespoons)
- Dijon mustard (1 teaspoon)
- Salt and pepper to taste

Serving Size:
4 servings
Preparation Time:
15 minutes

1. In a large bowl, combine julienned apples, shredded cabbage, and shredded carrots.

2. In a small bowl, whisk together Greek yogurt, honey, lemon juice, Dijon mustard, salt, and pepper.

3. Pour the dressing over the slaw and toss gently to combine.

4. Serve this PCOS-friendly Apple Slaw chilled.

Swiss Chard Quiche

Swiss Chard Quiche offers a tasty and nutrient-packed option with Swiss chard providing essential vitamins and minerals. This quiche is a good source of protein and can be a satisfying meal.

Ingredients:
- Swiss chard (2 cups, chopped)
- Eggs (4)
- Milk (1 cup)
- Feta cheese (1/2 cup, crumbled)
- Parmesan cheese (1/4 cup, grated)
- Cherry tomatoes (1/2 cup, halved)
- Olive oil (1 tablespoon)
- Salt and pepper to taste

Serving Size:
4 servings
Cooking Time:
40 minutes

Instructions:

1. Before you start cooking, heat the oven to 375°F (190°C).

2. In a pan, sauté chopped Swiss chard in olive oil until wilted.

3. In a bowl, whisk together eggs, milk, crumbled feta cheese, grated Parmesan cheese, salt, and pepper.

4. Pour the egg mixture into a greased pie dish.

5. Add sautéed Swiss chard and halved cherry tomatoes on top.

6. Bake for 30-35 minutes or until the quiche is set and golden.

7. Serve and enjoy this Swiss Chard Quiche warm.

Grab 'n' Go Egg Muffins

Grab 'n' Go Egg Muffins offer a convenient and protein-packed option. Eggs provide essential nutrients and protein, which may contribute to improved satiety and blood sugar control.

Ingredients:
- Eggs (6)
- Spinach (1 cup, chopped)
- Cherry tomatoes (1/2 cup, diced)
- Feta cheese (1/4 cup, crumbled)
- Milk (1/4 cup)
- Olive oil (1 tablespoon)
- Salt and pepper to taste

Serving Size:
6 servings
Cooking Time:
20 minutes

1. Preheat the oven to 375°F (190°C).

2. In a bowl, whisk together eggs, chopped spinach, diced cherry tomatoes, crumbled feta cheese, milk, salt, and pepper.

3. Grease a muffin tin with olive oil.

4. Pour the egg mixture into each muffin cup.

5. Bake for 15-18 minutes or until the egg muffins are set.

6. Allow to cool slightly before removing from the muffin tin.

7. Serve these PCOS-friendly Grab 'n' Go Egg Muffins warm or refrigerate them for later use.

Main Course Recipes

Keto Pizza

Keto Pizza offers a low-carb alternative to traditional pizza, making it suitable for PCOS patients aiming to manage their carbohydrate intake. The recipe provides a source of healthy fats and protein.

Ingredients:
- Cauliflower (2 cups, riced)
- Mozzarella cheese (1 cup, shredded)
- Almond flour (1/4 cup)
- Eggs (2)
- Olive oil (1 tablespoon)
- Tomato sauce (1/2 cup, sugar-free)
- Cheese (1/2 cup, shredded, for topping)
- Toppings of choice (e.g., veggies, pepperoni, etc.)

Serving Size:

2 servings

Cooking Time:

25 minutes

Instructions:

1. Get the oven ready by setting it to 425°F (220°C) before you start cooking.

2. In a bowl, combine riced cauliflower, shredded mozzarella cheese, almond flour, and eggs.

3. Press the mixture onto a baking sheet to form a crust.

4. Brush the crust with olive oil and bake for 15 minutes.

5. Remove from the oven, add tomato sauce, cheese, and desired toppings.

6. Bake for an additional 10 minutes or until the cheese is melted and bubbly.

7. Serve this PCOS-friendly Keto Pizza hot.

Healthy Chicken Nuggets

Healthy Chicken Nuggets provide a lean protein option with less processed ingredients compared to traditional nuggets. The recipe supports a balanced diet for PCOS patients.

Ingredients:

- Chicken breasts (2, boneless and skinless)

- Almond flour (1 cup)

- Parmesan cheese (1/2 cup, grated)

- Garlic powder (1 teaspoon)

- Paprika (1 teaspoon)

- Salt and pepper to taste

- Eggs (2, beaten)

- Olive oil (2 tablespoons, for baking)

Serving Size:

4 servings

Cooking Time:

20 minutes

Instructions:

1. Warm up the oven by setting it to 400°F (200°C) before you begin cooking.

2. Cut chicken breasts into bite-sized nuggets.

3. In a bowl, mix almond flour, grated Parmesan cheese, garlic powder, paprika, salt, and pepper.

4. Dip each chicken nugget into beaten eggs, then coat with the almond flour mixture.

5. Place the nuggets on a baking sheet lined with parchment paper.

6. Drizzle olive oil over the nuggets.

7. Bake for 15-18 minutes or until golden brown and cooked through.

8. Serve these PCOS-friendly Healthy Chicken Nuggets hot.

Vegetable Stews

Vegetable Stews offer a nutrient-rich and fiber-packed option with various vegetables. This recipe supports a balanced diet and may contribute to improved blood sugar control.

Ingredients:

- Mixed vegetables (e.g., carrots, celery, bell peppers, zucchini) (3 cups, chopped)
- Vegetable broth (4 cups)
- Onion (1, diced)
- Garlic (2 cloves, minced)
- Tomato paste (2 tablespoons)
- Olive oil (2 tablespoons)
- Herbs and spices (e.g., thyme, rosemary, bay leaves)
- Salt and pepper to taste

Serving Size:
4 servings
Cooking Time:
30 minutes

Instructions:

1. In a pot, sauté diced onion and minced garlic in olive oil until softened.

2. Add chopped mixed vegetables and continue to sauté for 5 minutes.

3. Stir in tomato paste and herbs/spices.

4. Pour in vegetable broth, bring to a boil, then simmer for 20-25 minutes.

5. Sprinkle some salt and pepper according to your taste.

6. Serve this PCOS-friendly Vegetable Stew hot.

Creamy Bell Pepper Soup

Creamy Bell Pepper Soup offers a flavorful and nutrient-dense option with bell peppers providing antioxidants and vitamin C. The soup is low in carbs and can be a good choice for PCOS patients managing their carbohydrate intake.

Ingredients:
- Bell peppers (4, red or yellow, roasted and peeled)
- Onion (1, diced)
- Garlic (2 cloves, minced)
- Vegetable broth (4 cups)
- Olive oil (2 tablespoons)
- Almond milk (1 cup)
- Salt and pepper to taste
- Fresh basil (for garnish)

Serving Size:

4 servings

Cooking Time:

30 minutes

Instructions:

1. Roast bell peppers, peel and chop.

2. In a pot, sauté diced onion and minced garlic in olive oil until softened.

3. Add chopped roasted bell peppers and vegetable broth. Simmer for 15-20 minutes.

4. Blend the mixture until smooth, then return to the pot.

5. Stir in almond milk and season with salt and pepper.

6. Garnish with fresh basil before serving.

7. Serve this and enjoy!

Skillet Chicken Breast with Broccoli Mash

Skillet Chicken Breast with Broccoli Mash offers a protein-packed meal with lean chicken breast and nutrient-rich broccoli. The recipe supports a balanced diet for PCOS patients and is low in carbs.

Ingredients:
- Chicken breasts (2, boneless and skinless)
- Broccoli (2 cups, florets)
- Chicken broth (1/2 cup)
- Garlic (2 cloves, minced)
- Olive oil (2 tablespoons)
- Salt and pepper to taste
- Lemon wedges (for serving)

Serving Size:

2 servings

Cooking Time:

25 minutes

Instructions:

1. Season chicken breasts with salt and pepper.

2. In a skillet, heat olive oil and cook chicken breasts until golden and cooked through.

3. In a separate pot, steam broccoli until tender.

4. Mash steamed broccoli and add minced garlic, chicken broth, salt, and pepper.

5. Serve the chicken breasts over the broccoli mash.

6. Squeeze lemon wedges over the dish before serving.

7. Serve this PCOS-friendly Skillet Chicken Breast with Broccoli Mash hot.

Chicken with Sweet Potatoes, Apples, and Brussels Sprouts

Chicken with Sweet Potatoes, Apples, and Brussels Sprouts provides a well-rounded and balanced meal with lean protein from chicken, complex carbohydrates from sweet potatoes, and fiber from Brussels sprouts. This recipe supports a nutrient-dense and PCOS-friendly diet.

Ingredients:
- Chicken thighs (4, bone-in and skin-on)
- Sweet potatoes (2, peeled and diced)
- Apples (2, cored and sliced)
- Brussels sprouts (1 pound, halved)
- Olive oil (3 tablespoons)
- Maple syrup (2 tablespoons)
- Dijon mustard (1 tablespoon)
- Garlic powder (1 teaspoon)
- Salt and pepper to taste
- Fresh thyme (for garnish)

Serving Size:

4 servings

Cooking Time:

45 minutes

Instructions:

1. Before you start cooking, heat the oven to 400°F (200°C).

2. In a bowl, stir together olive oil, maple syrup, Dijon mustard, garlic powder, salt, and pepper.

3. Place chicken thighs, diced sweet potatoes, sliced apples, and halved Brussels sprouts on a baking sheet.

4. Brush the chicken and vegetables with the olive oil mixture.

5. Bake for 35-40 minutes or until the chicken is cooked through and the vegetables are tender.

6. Garnish with fresh thyme before serving.

7. Serve this PCOS-friendly Chicken with Sweet Potatoes, Apples, and Brussels Sprouts.

Zucchini Noodles with Avocado Pesto Shrimp

Zucchini Noodles with Avocado Pesto Shrimp offers a low-carb alternative with zucchini noodles and nutrient-rich avocado. This recipe provides healthy fats and lean protein, supporting a PCOS-friendly diet.

Ingredients:
- Zucchini (4, spiralized into noodles)
- Shrimp (1 pound, peeled and deveined)
- Avocado (1, ripe)
- Basil leaves (1 cup)
- Garlic (2 cloves)
- Pine nuts (1/4 cup)
- Olive oil (3 tablespoons)
- Lemon juice (2 tablespoons)
- Salt and pepper to taste
- Cherry tomatoes (for garnish)

Serving Size:

4 servings

Cooking Time:

20 minutes

Instructions:

1. Turn zucchini into noodles using a spiralizer.

2. In a blender, combine avocado, basil, garlic, pine nuts, olive oil, lemon juice, salt, and pepper to make the pesto.

3. Sauté shrimp in a pan until cooked.

4. Toss zucchini noodles with avocado pesto and top with cooked shrimp.

5. Garnish with cherry tomatoes.

6. Serve these PCOS-friendly Zucchini Noodles with Avocado Pesto Shrimp immediately.

Sheet Pan Salmon and Potatoes

Sheet Pan Salmon and Potatoes provide a convenient and well-balanced meal with omega-3 fatty acids from salmon and complex carbohydrates from potatoes. This recipe supports a nutrient-dense and PCOS-friendly diet.

Ingredients:

- Salmon fillets (4)

- Potatoes (4, diced)

- Broccoli florets (2 cups)

- Olive oil (3 tablespoons)

- Garlic powder (1 teaspoon)

- Paprika (1 teaspoon)

- Lemon (1, sliced)

- Salt and pepper to taste

Serving Size:

4 servings

Cooking Time:

30 minutes

Instructions:

1. Preheat the oven to 400°F (200°C).

2. Place salmon fillets, diced potatoes, and broccoli florets on a sheet pan.

3. Drizzle with olive oil and sprinkle with garlic powder, paprika, salt, and pepper.

4. Toss to coat evenly and arrange lemon slices on top.

5. Bake for 20-25 minutes or until salmon is cooked through.

6. Serve this PCOS-friendly Sheet Pan Salmon and Potatoes hot.

Sweet and Sticky Orange Cauliflower

Sweet and Sticky Orange Cauliflower offers a flavorful and plant-based option with cauliflower as a low-carb alternative. This recipe provides fiber and is suitable for PCOS patients aiming to manage carbohydrate intake.

Ingredients:

- Cauliflower (1 head, cut into florets)
- Cornstarch (1/2 cup)
- Soy sauce (1/4 cup)
- Orange juice (1/4 cup)
- Honey (2 tablespoons)
- Rice vinegar (2 tablespoons)
- Garlic (2 cloves, minced)
- Ginger (1 teaspoon, grated)
- Sesame seeds (for garnish)
- Green onions (for garnish)

Serving Size:

4 servings

Cooking Time:

30 minutes

Instructions:

1. Preheat the oven to 400°F (200°C).

2. Toss cauliflower florets in cornstarch and bake until crispy.

3. In a saucepan, mix soy sauce, orange juice, honey, rice vinegar, minced garlic, and grated ginger. Simmer until thickened.

4. Toss baked cauliflower in the orange sauce.

5. Garnish with sesame seeds and green onions.

6. Serve this PCOS-friendly Sweet and Sticky Orange Cauliflower hot.

Honey Glazed Salmon

Honey Glazed Salmon provides omega-3 fatty acids and a touch of natural sweetness from honey. This recipe supports a balanced diet for PCOS patients.

Ingredients:
- Salmon fillets (4)
- Honey (1/4 cup)
- Soy sauce (2 tablespoons)
- Garlic (2 cloves, minced)
- Ginger (1 teaspoon, grated)
- Olive oil (2 tablespoons)
- Lemon juice (1 tablespoon)
- Sesame seeds (for garnish)
- Green onions (for garnish)

Serving Size:
4 servings
Cooking Time:
20 minutes

Instructions:

1. Preheat the oven to 400°F (200°C).

2. In a bowl, whisk together honey, soy sauce, minced garlic, grated ginger, olive oil, and lemon juice.

3. Place salmon fillets on a baking sheet and brush with the honey glaze.

4. Bake for 12-15 minutes or until salmon is cooked through.

5. Garnish with sesame seeds and green onions.

6. Serve this PCOS-friendly Honey Glazed Salmon hot.

Meal Plan

Week 1:

Day 1:

- Breakfast: Protein Waffles with Peanut Butter and Banana

- Lunch: Yogurt Bowl with Granola and Berries

- Dinner: Creamy Tomato Baked Fish

- Snack: Trail Mix

- Dessert: Chocolate Chia Pudding

Day 2:

- Breakfast: Smoothie with Greek Yogurt, Frozen Fruit, and Spinach

- Lunch: Spinach Chicken Poppers

- Dinner: Zuppa Toscana

- Snack: Guacamole

- Dessert: Banana Bread

Day 3:

- Breakfast: Cereal with Whole Milk, Turkey Bacon, Nuts, and Fruit

- Lunch: Prepared Greek Yogurt Cup with Nut/Granola Bar and Banana

- Dinner: Honey Glazed Salmon

- Snack: Zucchini Chips
- Dessert: Berry Delight

Week 2:

Day 4:

- Breakfast: Protein Oats with Chopped Nuts and Fruit
- Lunch: Chicken Collard Wraps
- Dinner: Slow Cooked Beef and Broccoli
- Snack: Apple (or Any Fruit) with Nut Butter
- Dessert: Ginger Cookies

Day 5:

- Breakfast: Smoothie with Kefir, Avocado, and Flaxseed
- Lunch: Beet, Goat Cheese, Broccoli Salad
- Dinner: Harvest Chicken Chili
- Snack: Zucchini Noodles with Avocado Pesto Shrimp
- Dessert: Chai Tea Frozen Yogurt

Day 6:

- Breakfast: Bento with Boiled Eggs, Yogurt, Nuts, Fruit, Cucumber, and Muffin
- Lunch: Guacamole Chicken Salad
- Dinner: Shrimp Fried Rice
- Snack: Guacamole
- Dessert: Creamy Mango Pineapple Smoothie

Week 3:

Day 7:

- Breakfast: Toast with Avocado and Egg
- Lunch: Sweet Potato Noodle Salad
- Dinner: Creamy Cauliflower Soup
- Snack: Supercharged Green Smoothie
- Dessert: Chai Tea Frozen Yogurt

Day 8:

- Breakfast: Muffin with Boiled Eggs and Trail Mix
- Lunch: Quinoa Salad with Roasted Vegetables
- Dinner: Zucchini Noodles with Avocado Pesto Shrimp

- Snack: Zucchini Chips
- Dessert: Avocado Berry Fertility Smoothie

Day 9:

- Breakfast: Prepared Greek Yogurt Cup with Nut/Granola Bar and Banana
- Lunch: Chicken Collard Wraps
- Dinner: Sheet Pan Salmon and Potatoes
- Snack: Trail Mix
- Dessert: Chocolate Mud Cake

Conclusion

You have reached the end of this book, but not the end of your journey. You have learned a lot about PCOS and nutrition, and you have tried many delicious and nutritious recipes. You have also followed Agnes' story, and seen how she transformed her PCOS and her life with the help of this book.

But this book is not the final destination. This marks the start of a fresh journey. An adventure that will take you to places you never imagined. Places where you will feel healthy, happy, and hopeful. Places where you will achieve your dreams, whether it is losing weight, clearing your skin, improving your mood, or getting pregnant. This book is not a one-time read. It is a lifelong companion. A companion that will support you, guide you and inspire you. A companion that will remind you that you are not alone, that you are not a victim, that you are a warrior.

This book is not a cookbook. It is a manifesto. A manifesto that will empower you, challenge you and motivate you. A manifesto that will show you that you can overcome PCOS and reclaim your health and your happiness. This book is not just for you. It is for every woman who has PCOS, knows someone who has PCOS, or cares about someone who has PCOS. It is for every woman who wants to make a difference, not only in her own life but in the lives of others.

This book is for you, Agnes, and all the women like you. It is time to celebrate your achievements, share your stories, and spread your wisdom. It is time to join the easy PCOS diet cookbook community.